DASH Diet

Overcome Hypertension, Lose Weight, and Experience a New Level of Health

Thomas Rohmer

Disclaimer:

This guide has been created for informational and reference
purposes only. The author, publisher, and any other
affiliated parties cannot be held in any way accountable for
any personal injuries or damage allegedly resulting from the
information contained herein, or from any misuse of such
guidance. Although strict measures have been taken to
provide accurate information, the parties involved with the
creation and publication of this guide take no responsibility
for any issues that many arise from alleged discrepancies
contained herein. It is strongly recommended that you
consult a physician, personal trainer, and nutritionist prior
to commencing this or any other workout or diet plan. This
guide is not a substitute for professional personal guidance
from a qualified medical professional. If you feel pain or
discomfort at any point during exercises contained herein,
cease the activity immediately and seek medical guidance.

Before You Begin:

Get the Latest Scoop on the Most Cutting Edge Info on Health & Fitness!

As thanks for picking up this book, I'd love to offer you the chance to maximize your results by getting exclusive info on health and fitness.

You'll be the first to know when I publish new books, and you'll receive exclusive content on health and fitness that I only share with people on my list.

Simply visit the link directly below and get started on the path to the healthiest version of yourself today!

https://rohmerfitness.lpages.co/kindle-sign-up/

Table of Contents

Introduction:

It's the 21st century and we've made great advances in things like technology and medicine. However, when it comes to our health, we seem to have taken a step back. People today are ridden with things like Type 2 Diabetes and cardiovascular disease among other things. Why is it that we've made such great improvements in certain areas like technology, yet the obesity rate continues to increase?

It comes down to the wrong information. We are constantly being sold on gimmicks like weight loss pills and other sketchy powders and potions that are supposed to magically help us lose weight, get our blood pressure in check, and make us healthy again. But clearly none of those things are coming true. We try diet after diet in the hopes that it'll finally be the answer, and all we end up with is disappointment.

Luckily this all changes for you today. In this book, you'll discover what has been named as the best diet multiple years in a row. It's not some gimmicky overnight fix. Instead it's something that actually works.

I'm talking about the DASH diet here. This nutritional approach will finally allow you to lose weight and get your health back. Not only that, but it isn't that hard of a diet to follow! Most diets have confusing rules like you can only eat at a certain time or they force you to eat certain foods.

That won't be the case with the DASH diet. In this book, you'll learn about all of the ins and outs of the DASH diet.

You'll understand all of the health benefits you can expect to gain from following this eating plan. You'll even learn how to use exercise to further benefit your nutrition plan. And finally you'll be given a step-by-step process along with a 14-day sample meal plan to help you get started on the right foot with the DASH diet. Let's dive in and get started...

Chapter 1: What is the DASH Diet?

The DASH diet stands for dietary approaches to stop hypertension, and the main goal of the diet is to do just that—stop hypertension. Hypertension is high blood pressure, and it's something that affects more people than you might think. According to the CDC, high blood pressure affects nearly 75 million American adults (1). That's nearly 1 out of every 3 people!

And of the people who do have high blood pressure, approximately half of those people don't have it under control (2)! You might be wondering why having high blood pressure is such a big deal. Hypertension can lead to heart and kidney disease, stroke, and even blindness.

And with the way most people eat, it starts to become much more apparent as to why our blood pressure is getting out of control. The standard American diet (which stands for SAD) consists mostly of processed foods, artificially sweetened foods, red meats, foods high in salt, and take out food at least once per week, but possibly more often than that (3).

In addition to that, 1 out of every 3 Americans are either overweight or obese (4), and show signs of metabolic syndrome. Metabolic syndrome is characterized by having excess weight, especially around the stomach/abdomen area, high blood pressure, slightly higher blood sugar, and problems with cholesterol and the number of triglycerides in the blood.

So clearly something needs to change in regards to the way that most people are eating nowadays. The DASH diet cannot only help you lower your blood pressure, but it can also help you maintain a healthy bodyweight. The primary focus of the DASH diet is to help you eat the right amount of fruits, vegetables, whole grains, and low-fat dairy products.

These types of foods are high in fiber, contain a moderate amount of fat, and are rich in potassium, calcium, and magnesium. Consuming more of these nutrients and minerals will help you to start seeing some improvements in your overall health by doing things like lowering blood pressure, improving digestion, and staying fuller for a longer period of time.

The DASH diet also will reduce salt intake, saturated fat, processed foods, eliminate trans fat, and sweets. With the DASH diet eating plan, it's not just about what foods you're going to be consuming. Equally as important are what foods you're going to drastically reduce or eliminate altogether.

You can eat all of the nutrient-rich foods that you want such as fruits and vegetables, and that's great! However, the thing you have to remember is that you can quickly offset the benefits of those healthy foods by eating junk. Consuming processed foods, salty foods, or foods that aren't that healthy will do you no good and cause you to take a step back in your quest to become a healthier individual.

So don't think of this diet strictly in terms of what you'll be eating because what you eliminate from your diet will be equally as important to your success with the diet plan.

Chapter 2: Best Foods to Eat on the DASH Diet

The following are the best foods you can eat while on the DASH diet. These are foods that are high in fiber, magnesium, potassium, and other vitamins and minerals. This is not meant to be a comprehensive list, rather this is meant to give you some good ideas for what you should be eating while on the DASH diet.

Vegetables

While following the DASH diet, you should be consuming around 4-5 servings of vegetables per day. We all know that vegetables are good for us and that they are very healthy foods, yet I think few of us realize just how healthy vegetables really are:

- Eating vegetables regularly can help to reduce the risk of heart disease and stroke (5).

- It can help protect you against certain types of cancer (6).

- Vegetables are low in calories and high in fiber. This means that you can eat as much of them as you want and not have to worry about overeating. And the fiber will help to keep you fuller for a longer period of time as well as ensure proper bowel movements.

- Vegetables are very nutrient dense, meaning that they contain a lot of nutrients even though they're low in overall calories. Something like a candy bar, on the other hand, isn't nutrient dense. It contains a lot of calories, but it has very few nutrients.

- Folic acid: folic acid helps the body to create red blood cells. Red blood cells are necessary for transporting oxygen throughout your body. Getting proper amounts of folic acid is especially important for pregnant women or women who plan on becoming pregnant to ensure proper fetal development.

- Vegetables are rich in so many vitamins and minerals! Vegetables contain high amounts of vitamin A, C, potassium, iron, magnesium, and calcium.

Here's a list of vegetables that you should consume on the DASH diet:

- Sweet potatoes
- Tomatoes
- Squash
- Spinach
- Potatoes
- Lima Beans
- Kale
- Green Beans
- Peas
- Collard Greens
- Mustard Greens
- Broccoli
- Cauliflower
- Carrots

Fruits

Just like vegetables, fruits are very good for you and will provide you with many of the same vitamins and minerals that vegetables will. Unfortunately, fruits sometimes get a bad reputation because they contain fructose, which is a type of sugar. The thing is though that fructose is a natural sugar, not a processed sugar, and the benefits you'll receive from eating fruits far outweighs the fact that they contain some sugar in them.

While following the DASH diet eating plan, you'll want to consume 4-5 servings of fruit per day. Here are some of the amazing benefits of eating fruit:

- Fruits contain low amounts of sodium, calories, and fat.

- Similar to vegetables, fruit is very nutrient dense. So basically you'll be getting a good bang-for-your-buck when it comes to getting the most nutrients for the least amount of calories. Eating rich nutrient dense foods is critical for your success with the DASH diet.

- Fruits can help to lower cholesterol levels as well as reduce the risk for heart disease (7).

- Additionally, fruits contain high amounts of vitamin A and C, potassium, magnesium, folic acid, and fiber.

- Fruits also contain high amounts of water, which will help to keep your body hydrated.

Here's a list of fruits you should consume on the DASH diet:

- Raisins
- Blueberries
- Raspberries
- Strawberries
- Peaches
- Pineapples
- Melons

- Grapes
- Apples
- Apricots
- Bananas
- Dates
- Oranges
- Grapefruit
- Mangoes
- Tangerines

Dairy

While on the DASH diet eating plan, you should be
consuming around 2-3 servings of dairy per day. It's
important to note that you'll want to be eating low-fat dairy.
The DASH diet limits certain types of fat intake, and
consuming large amounts of fat through dairy isn't ideal,
especially if it can be avoided in the first place. Here are
some of the key benefits of consuming dairy in your diet:

- Dairy is high in protein. Protein is one of three
  macronutrients (carbs and fat being the other two),
  and it's responsible for aiding in many of your body's
  functions. One of the main things protein does is
  rebuild and repair tissue.

  It's an important building block for muscle, bone,
  skin, cartilage, and blood. It's also needed for the
  growth of hair and nails. So needless to say, protein is
  a very critical nutrient regardless if you're looking to
  pack on muscle or not.

- Dairy is rich in calcium. When you think of strong
  bones, what do you think of? You probably think of
  some kid or adult drinking a glass of milk. We've
  really been bombarded with the fact that milk (and
  other dairy products for that matter) is good for
  strong bones, and it really is so true! This is all

because of calcium. Calcium is necessary for maintaining bone mass in the body, which helps to support the skeleton.

The thing is though we lose a lot of calcium through normal bodily processes in the kidneys and colon. Calcium is also used in muscle and nerve functions as well. And if we don't supply our bodies with enough calcium, then our bodies will start to pull the stored calcium in our bones in order to carry out its normal everyday functions.

This is why it's so important to be able to get the proper amount of calcium. It's not just used for our bones, but for many other necessary functions of our bodies. If we're not consuming an adequate amount of calcium, then that's when our bones will take a hit.

They'll start to become more brittle and frail. This can then lead to osteoporosis. Approximately 44 million Americans suffer from osteoporosis or low bone mass, and 55% of Americans over the age of 50 have osteoporosis (8). Osteoporosis will lead to more bone and hip fractures, which will inhibit mobility along with making it much harder to follow a diet plan such as DASH.

The following are some good sources of dairy that you can eat. Remember to go with the low-fat option when possible:

- Skim Milk
- 1% Milk
- Low-Fat Cheese
- Low-Fat Cottage Cheese
- Low-Fat Yogurt

Meats, Poultry, and Fish

You'll also be consuming some meat on the DASH diet plan. Meat isn't as heavily emphasized as some of the other food groups, such as fruits and vegetables however, it's still an important part of the diet regime. You'll want to consume around 1-2 servings of meat, poultry, and/or fish per day.

When consuming these meats, you'll want to make sure that you're going with lean meats. Additionally, be sure to trim away any visible fat from the meat that you can. Finally, the way you cook and prepare the meat matters as well. Avoid frying the food as this will make it have excess fat that isn't necessary. Instead, you'll want to broil, roast, or poach the meat.

This is the healthiest way to prepare your food. On a side note, when you're preparing poultry, remove the skin. Getting rid of the skin will help to remove more of the fat content contained in the chicken. Here are some of the benefits of consuming meat, poultry, and fish:

- High in protein: Similar to dairy products, any meat that you consume will have a good amount of protein in it. As mentioned earlier, this is important for repairing muscle tissue, growing hair and nails, as well as being an important building block for skin, bone, cartilage, and blood.

- Lean meats also contain a high amount of magnesium. Magnesium is critical for the proper functioning of hundreds of enzymes. Research has shown that magnesium can help to reduce blood pressure with individuals who are suffering from hypertension (9).

  It can also help with type 2 diabetes (10). And it can even help to fight depression (11). Fortunately, the DASH diet will allow you to consume plenty of magnesium, not just from lean meats, but from other food sources as well. Here's a list of lean meats that you can consume:

- Poultry
- Fish
- Bison
- Venison
- Beef

Nuts, Seeds, and Dried Beans

You'll want to consume 3 servings of various nuts, seeds, and dried beans per week on the DASH diet. You'll be eating quite a bit less of this food group compared to some of the other food groups, and it's for a good reason. Nuts are comprised mostly of fat.

Yes, there are good types of fat and bad types of fat (more on this later), however fat contains 9 calories per gram. On the other hand, protein and carbs only contain 4 calories per gram of food. This means that you'll be consuming over twice the amount of calories for the same amount of food if you're consuming fat. Those calories can add up rather quickly, and this is something we want to be aware of.

That's why you'll only be consuming 3 servings per week of these different nuts, seeds, and dried beans. As I just mentioned though, there is such a thing as good fat and bad fat. Bad fats would be something like trans fat and saturated fat. Excessive amounts of these types of fat have been shown to increase the risk for heart disease as well as other health problems (12).

Nuts and seeds, on the other hand, contain mono and polyunsaturated fats. These are a healthy type of fat that can help to lower your risk of heart disease by decreasing your low-density lipoproteins (LDL) and maintaining your high-density lipoproteins (HDL). Your LDL's are the bad type of cholesterol, and your HDL's are the good kind of cholesterol.

Of course, this idea of there being a good type of fat might be hard for you to grasp at first. Just like myself, you probably grew up learning that fat is bad for you. Intuitively this makes sense because we can see how excess fat on our bodies is bad for us so it naturally makes sense that consuming fat is harmful. However, this couldn't be further from the truth.

The reality is that consuming too many calories overall from all three macronutrients (protein, carbs, and fat) is bad for us and that's what leads to weight gain. Yes, certain types of fat should be limited or avoided altogether (such as saturated or trans fat), but that's not to say that all fat is bad for you because that simply isn't the case. Here are some of the benefits of consuming nuts, seeds, and dried beans:

- They are a rich source of energy. As I talked about earlier, fat contains 9 calories per gram. This can be dangerous if overeaten, however you have to remember why we're eating food in the first place—to get energy! Our body needs daily energy to maintain itself and carry out its daily functions.

  And where do our bodies get that needed energy? It gets it from the foods that we eat of course! Eating nuts is a great way to give our bodies a solid source of calories if we need to consume more. Just be careful not to overdo it!

- Contain healthy amounts of magnesium and fiber. Are you starting to notice a common theme here? Many of the foods you'll be consuming on the DASH diet are rich in magnesium! It's such a key mineral for getting and staying healthy, especially if you have hypertension.

Not only that, but nuts, seeds, and dried beans contain fiber. This is something that the typical American doesn't get enough of, and it's no wonder why so many people struggle with digestive issues.

- Finally, this food group surprisingly contains a good amount of protein. This is something you might not expect at first, but it's certainly true. For example, one serving of almonds contains 6 grams of protein! So not only will you be consuming healthy fats when you eat nuts, but you'll also be getting a decent amount of protein as well.

Now that you know the benefits of this food group, here's a list of some different kinds of them you can eat on the DASH diet (of course always go with the unsalted version whenever possible):

- Almonds
- Hazelnuts
- Mixed Nuts
- Peanuts
- Walnuts
- Sunflower Seeds
- Natural Peanut Butter
- Natural Almond Butter
- Kidney Beans
- Lentils
- Split Peas

Fats and Oils

Fats and oils are another essential part of the DASH diet. Again fats have gotten a bad reputation over the years, but it isn't all justified. The same goes for oils. When you think of oily food, what do you typically think of? Probably something that's greasy, fried, contains a lot of fat, and is unhealthy for you right?

Well yes, some oils are really bad for you. However, not all oils are as bad as they might seem. As I mentioned earlier, there are good fats and bad fats. You want to limit bad fats from your diet such as saturated fat and trans fat.

And you'll want to consume more healthy fats like mono and polyunsaturated fats. That's why you'll want to use oils that contain healthy fats like mono and polyunsaturated fats. The best kind of oil you can use for is olive oil. This is a healthy type of oil that contains a good amount of monounsaturated fat.

Canola oil can be a good option to use as well due to its high monounsaturated fat content as well, but use olive oil when you can as a first option. In terms of how much fats and oils you should be consuming, look to get roughly 2 servings of fats and oils per day. Here are some of the benefits of consuming fats and oils:

- Regulation of body temperature: Fats are important for regulating your body temperature and helping to keep it at a normal and healthy range.

- Good for brain health: non-water soluble vitamins such as vitamins A, D, E, and K need fat to get absorbed and transported by the body. These vitamins are critical for a properly functioning brain. Not only that, but your brain is made up of close to 60% fat (13)! So needless to say, it's quite important that you get an adequate amount of fat in your diet.

- Source of energy: fat can be stored in the body for later use, however it can also be used as a more primary source of energy if the body is low on carbohydrates or low on calories.

- Healthy skin and hair: Fat can help to make skin and hair appear soft, silky, and smooth due to its protective qualities. Without this protection from fat, harmful chemicals would be able to more easily enter the body through the skin.

Whole Grains

On the DASH eating plan, you're going to want to consume 6-8 servings of whole grains per day. It's very important to note that you'll want to be consuming whole grains here and not refined grains. Refined grains are more processed than whole grains and thus lose vitamins, minerals, and fiber during the process.

Whole grains, on the other hand, contain more vitamins and fiber, which is key to keeping you fuller longer. Whole grains still contain all three parts of the grain, which are the bran, germ, and endosperm.

When refined grains get processed, they're stripped of the bran and germ, which contain many key nutrients. Not only that, but whole grains are rich in things such as thiamin, riboflavin, niacin, and folate. These are part of the B vitamins complex. B vitamins are important for many different things including:
- Making new cells
- Red cell production
- Increase in HDL cholesterol (which is the good kind of cholesterol)
- Preventing memory loss
- Keeping depression at bay

Here's a list of acceptable whole grains should you eat while on the DASH diet:

- Whole-wheat pasta
- Whole-wheat bread
- Brown rice
- Whole-grain cereal

Chapter 3: Foods You'll Want to Limit on the DASH Diet

One of the things I really like about the DASH diet is that it doesn't entirely forbid you to eat the foods you love. I've seen plenty of people start a new diet plan only to fail a few short weeks later when they couldn't handle the misery anymore. Here's how it usually goes down:

1. You start a new diet and get all excited about it.
2. You immediately go cold turkey and cut all junk food from your diet.
3. For the first few days and maybe even weeks, things go pretty smoothly.
4. Then something comes up, like your best friend's birthday party for example.
5. While at the party, you do your best to stay on track with your diet plan.
6. You see everyone around you having a good time and eating as they please.
7. You really can't handle it anymore so you tell yourself you've been good and one piece of cake can't hurt that bad right?
8. You eat the piece of cake and then proceed to binge eat everything in sight.
9. Later that night you feel guilty for binge eating junk food and feel disgusted with yourself.
10. You also wonder if you'll ever be able to get the hang of this diet thing.
11. Then a few days or weeks later when you're feeling better about yourself, you start a new diet and the cycle repeats itself.

You see the problem in the above scenario isn't the fact that the person ate a slice of birthday cake. The reality is that one piece of cake, one brownie, one bowl of ice cream, etc. *can't* completely wreck your diet in one fell swoop. What does ruin your diet is when you feel guilty for eating something you feel like you shouldn't of.

These feelings of guilt then cause you to say "screw it," which is when you'll proceed to binge eat anything your heart desires at that moment. And it's the binge eating that'll mess up your nutrition plan. Instead, a much better approach is to occasionally allow sweets or other treats in your diet from time to time.

Think about it, if it's in your diet plan to eat a small bowl of ice cream every three days, are you going to feel guilty when you eat that ice cream? No, you won't because it's part of the diet plan! On the flip side, if all junk food is forbidden under any circumstances, how are you going to feel if you eat a sweet treat? You'll feel horrible!

You'll feel like you cheated on your diet and that it's all over with. That, of course, isn't true, but at that moment, most people feel like complete failures. And this is one of the things I love most about the DASH diet. On the DASH diet eating plan, you're allowed to eat up to five servings of sweets per week.

This means that you won't have to completely give up your favorite sweet treats if you don't want to. The DASH diet is realistic about the fact that we're human. Seriously, who do you know of that could go the rest of their lives without eating another piece of junk food ever again? Probably no one! That's why the DASH diet is really not a diet as much as it's a lifestyle plan.

It's something that you'll easily be able to do for a very long time to come. This is great news when compared to other nutrition plans. Every day when you wake up, you think to yourself, "Dang another day of boring eating, I'm not sure how much longer I can handle this." And most people don't last long on boring diet plans that have them eating the same bland foods day in and day out.

With that being said, you'll of course want to limit certain food choices on the DASH diet. You can certainly include these things as part of your 5 servings of sweets per week, but be cautious not to overdo it. The servings and calories can add up rather quickly if you do! This list isn't meant to scare you into not eating any of these foods, but rather to help you better understand why they need to be limited in order for you to be successful with the DASH diet plan.

Processed foods:

Processed foods are made with certain ingredients that will extend the shelf life of those foods. On one hand, this seems great. It allows the expiration date of a food item to be extended longer so we can take a longer time to eat the food if we wish.

However, we have to take a step back and consider the harmful effects these ingredients can have on our bodies over the long haul. Here are some reasons why you'll want to limit the consumption of processed foods:

Empty calories: processed foods in most cases contain a lot of empty calories. Imagine eating broccoli for example. This vegetable is rich in a lot of key vitamins and nutrients that your body needs. It doesn't contain a lot of calories, and the calories that it does contain are jam-packed with healthy nutrients.

On the flip side, consider a processed food item such as a candy bar. The candy bar doesn't contain very many beneficial vitamins and minerals for our bodies. It also contains a lot of calories from simple sugars. That's why the calories from something like a candy bar are considered to be empty. They're providing your body with nothing useful that it needs.

So you'll likely be unable to get full and stay satisfied, meaning that you'll have to eat even more calories. This is why you must be cautious when eating processed foods. The calories won't do much to keep you full, and it can be very easy to overeat them.

High in trans fat and processed oils: Remember that on the DASH diet we are seeking to eliminate or greatly limit the amount of trans fat that we're consuming. Most processed foods contain quite a bit of trans fat and processed oils that we'll want to avoid. These kinds of fats are high in Omega-6 fatty acids.

Omega-6 fatty acids by themselves are not bad, however they can become a problem when consumed in excess compared to Omega-3 fatty acids. Omega-6 fatty acids cause our bodies to become inflamed. Excess inflammation can cause damage to our joints, impede recovery, and cause heart disease among other things (14).

This is why it's important to have a balance of Omega-3 fatty acids, which act as an anti-inflammatory in the body. The Omega-3 fatty acids can help to counteract the inflammation from the Omega-6 fatty acids.

Low in fiber: processed foods contain a low amount of fiber. Other foods like fruits and vegetables contain high amounts of fiber. As I've talked about earlier, fiber is not only important for our digestive health, but it's also very important for keeping us full for longer periods of time.

This is the real danger of eating too much processed foods. They don't fill you up very well, so you have to eat more of them to get full. This likely means that you'll eat more calories than you should have.

Contain simple carbohydrates: Some people think that you should avoid carbs at all costs, and it's easy to believe considering how bad of a reputation carbs have been getting lately. However, all of this hate on carbs isn't justified. There are good carbs and bad carbs.

Not all carbs are evil and should be avoided like the plague. There are two different kinds of carbohydrates—simple and complex. Simple carbs are carbs that are quickly broken down and processed by the body. This is a bad thing because the rapid breakdown leads to a spike in your insulin levels.

Insulin spikes can lead to food cravings at random times, and your body doesn't burn fat while your insulin levels are high (15).

Conversely, there are complex carbohydrates. These are carbs such as brown rice and sweet potatoes. These kinds of carbs are slower digesting carbs that will not cause spikes in your blood sugar levels. Complex carbs are considered to be a healthy carb that also contains many beneficial vitamins and nutrients.

Sodas:

Sodas should be severely limited if not completely eliminated on the DASH diet. Limiting or eliminating soda intake is one of the first steps I have people take to start losing weight. The reason is similar to why you'd want to limit your intake of processed foods. Sodas contain an excessive amount of sugar, high fructose corn syrup, and empty calories.

Unlike certain processed foods, I consider soda and candy to be the ultimate forms of empty calories because they literally contain only sugar. They provide absolutely zero nutrition that's beneficial for your body. Soda and candy will do nothing to keep you full, and they'll give you random cravings—not good at all!

Excessive amounts of sugar have been linked to many negative health effects such as increased fat mass, increased amount of triglycerides in the blood, insulin resistance, and increase in low-density lipoproteins (the bad form of cholesterol) among other things (16). So needless to say, soda is something you'll definitely want to watch out for.

The thing is sugar can be quite addicting (17), so how can you start to limit your soda intake if it's currently too high? I would avoid trying to quit cold turkey. Imagine if you've been drinking an average of two sodas per day for the last five years.

Is it really that likely you'll be able to walk away from it and never look back? Doubtful. Instead, you need to take a more steady approach. If for example, you're drinking 16 ounces of soda per day, then start off by pouring out 4 ounces of the soda and diluting the remaining 12 ounces with 4 ounces of water.

After doing that for a week, take another step forward by pouring out 8 ounces of soda and diluting the remaining 8 ounces of soda with 8 ounces of water. From there, once that week has finished, you can do 4 ounces of soda with 12 ounces of water. And then move completely away from it.

Sure it's tempting to want to go all out and eliminate soda completely in one fell swoop, but know yourself and be wise. If you think you'd be more successful by being patient and gradually easing yourself off of soda, then do that.

Juices and other artificially sweetened beverages

Wait what? I thought things like orange juice were good for you? Yes, if you took oranges, squeezed them, and only drank the juice that came directly from the oranges that would be ok.

However, most fruit juices and other artificially sweetened beverages aren't healthy options. The main reason why is because they are loaded with a bunch of excessive sugar. Most juices don't contain purely the sugar found in the fruits.

Most of the time, there's added sugar in the juices. Yes, these juices do contain a lot of vitamins such as vitamin A and C, however this doesn't make them a healthy drink option. In fact, this deceives people into thinking that it's a healthy choice when the truth is that it's not.

If you want to get more vitamin A and C in your diet, then eat more fruits and vegetables. You don't have to go out of your way by drinking more fruit juices to get more vitamins. Yes, it's easier to consume these vitamins by drinking them, but it comes at a cost. And that cost is excessive amounts of sugar.

As mentioned earlier, too much sugar in the diet has been shown to lead to health problems such as metabolic syndrome, certain types of cancer, and diabetes. In addition to that, sugar has been shown to be highly addictive, so you must be careful with how much you consume. It's certainly best to avoid the unnecessary sugar and get your vitamins and nutrients from whole food sources such as fruits and vegetables.

White Bread

On the DASH diet, you're going to consuming whole grains, such as whole-wheat bread. Something you'll want to avoid is white bread. On the surface, it might appear as if bread is bread so what's the big deal with white bread? Why do we want to avoid eating it whenever possible?

For starters, white bread is a simple carbohydrate. As I talked about earlier, simple carbs should be avoided in favor of complex carbs. Simple carbohydrates provide little nutritional value to your body, and they also cause rapid spikes in your blood sugar levels, which can lead to food cravings at random times throughout the day.

Not only that, but white bread ranks high on the glycemic index scale (GI scale for short). The GI scale measures how fast or slow different carbohydrates cause increases in blood glucose levels. The slower the carbohydrate increases blood glucose levels, the better it is, and thus the lower the score it'll receive on the glycemic index scale.

The scale ranges from 0-100, and basically what you need to know is that the closer a food item is to 0, the better it is for you. White bread has a GI score of 75 (18), which isn't good at all. It'll quickly raise blood sugar levels much faster than other carbohydrates will. That's why on the DASH diet, you'll be consuming whole grains, which rank much lower on the glycemic index scale. And you'll want to greatly limit or completely avoid carbs such as white bread.

French Fries

French fries are essentially the fried version of a potato. Now there's nothing wrong with a regular white potato or a sweet potato. However, when you take a potato and fry it, many things happen along the way that makes the food item unhealthy. For instance, when the food is being cooked, it's being fried in unhealthy oils.

This is going to drastically increase the amount of fat content in the food. Not only that but when you order fries from a fast food restaurant, what are they going to add to the fries? That's right, they're going to add salt. This will unnecessarily increase the amount of sodium in the food.

And as you learned from earlier, taking in too much sodium can cause hypertension, which is why you'll want to limit sodium intake on the DASH diet. Finally, fries are very easy

to over consume. Think about how long it takes you to eat a
potato or sweet potato. Now compare that to how long it
takes you to wolf down a side of medium fries from a fast
food restaurant.

And since these fries contain a lot of added fat, this means
that they contain an excessive amount of calories as well.
Plus you won't be eating the fries plain as they are, of course
you'll have to dip them in ketchup with contains high
fructose corn syrup and more sugar than you'd think. Fries
are definitely something you can overeat rather quickly, so
be very cautious of this food on the DASH diet.

Cookies, cakes, and other pastries

These sweet treats are another simple carbohydrate that
you'll want to watch out for. Their nutritional content is
made up primarily of refined sugars and other processed
ingredients. These foods usually contain shortening, which is
a type of solid fat that's high in saturated fat. This is one of
the bad types of fat that you'll want to limit whenever
possible. Yes, these foods are tasty, but be wary not to over
consume them as part of your 5 servings per week following
the nutritional plan.

Chapter 4: Health Benefits of the DASH Diet

Chances are good that you want to start the DASH diet eating plan because you want to improve your health. What health benefits can you expect to gain from following this nutrition plan? Well, quite a few things as it turns out.

The DASH diet has been voted to be the best diet 6 years in a row by U.S. News and World Report (19). Obviously there must be many great things about it to be able to uphold that type of a standard. Let's go ahead and jump into those benefits right now:

Health Benefit #1: Lowering of Cholesterol

Cholesterol is a waxy substance found in most of your body's tissues. It's mostly made in the liver, but cholesterol can also be found in foods such as eggs, butter, and cheese. When most people hear the word cholesterol, they think of something negative and unhealthy, but that actually isn't the case.

Cholesterol is necessary for the building of new cells. It only becomes a problem when the amount of cholesterol in the blood becomes too high. Most people don't realize that there are two different kinds of cholesterol— high-density lipoproteins (HDL's) and low-density lipoproteins (LDL's). Your high-density lipoproteins are your body's good type of cholesterol and it's responsible for carrying your LDL's to the liver to be disposed of, and it stops the build-up of LDL's in the arteries.

As you can probably already guess, low-density lipoproteins are your body's bad type of cholesterol, and LDL's stick to artery walls, narrow artery walls, and cause plaque build-up. In reality, if you're looking to lower your cholesterol levels, what you're actually wanting to do is decrease your bad cholesterol levels (aka your LDL's), and you're looking to increase the amount of good cholesterol (aka your HDL's).

The main way the DASH diet is going to work to lower your bad cholesterol levels is by controlling the foods you eat—specifically your fat intake in this case. When we eat a lot of high fatty foods, this can cause issues with our cholesterol levels if we're not careful. This is especially true if the fat content we're eating is saturated fat and trans fat.

These are unhealthy types of fat that'll be limited on the DASH eating plan. Once these types of fat are severely limited or eliminated completely, you won't be raising your low-density lipoprotein levels, but rather decreasing them. Not all fats will be completely eliminated on the DASH diet of course.

And the healthy fats that you'll be consuming will help to increase the good type of cholesterol in your body. Additionally, losing weight and exercising regularly will also help to increase the number of high-density lipoproteins in your body, which I'll talk more about later.

Health Benefit #2: Lowering Blood Pressure

This is considered to be the biggest benefit of the DASH diet considering that its name stands for dietary approaches to stop hypertension. But what exactly is blood pressure anyway? Why is lowering your blood pressure so important for your overall health and well being?

Your body needs oxygen and energy in order to properly function. Every time your heart beats, it pumps blood, which contains oxygen and other rich nutrients throughout your entire body. Your blood is carried throughout your body via blood vessels. Your blood pushes against the blood vessels. How hard your blood is pushing up against your blood vessels will determine your blood pressure.

The harder the blood pushes against the vessels, the higher your blood pressure will be. If your arteries are partially clogged with plaque, this will cause your body to have to work harder in order to keep pumping blood throughout your system.

This is why lowering your cholesterol levels can also help you to lower your blood pressure at the same time. Eventually, all of this extra stress and strain on your heart and vessels can lead to serious health problems such as a heart attack or stroke. Having hypertension is certainly no laughing matter, but how can you tell if you have high blood pressure in the first place?

The first thing you'll want to do is measure your blood pressure. You can get this measured by visiting your doctor, going to certain pharmacies, or even by buying your own blood pressure monitor at a store or online. The main thing you'll want to be aware of before taking your reading is that you haven't exercised for the past 2-3 hours.

Exercise increases blood flow in the body, and yes it's a very healthy thing to do, but it'll skew the reading not giving you an accurate picture of where your blood pressure actually is. Aside from that, be sure to follow these tips to ensure an accurate reading of your blood pressure:

1. Use a properly sized cuff that fits your arm size. Using an oversized cuff won't allow the machine to properly read your blood pressure, and using an undersized cuff will squeeze too tightly and be uncomfortable.

2. Sit in a chair with your arm resting on an armrest. You want your arm to be in a relaxed position instead of strained when the measurement is being taken.

3. Use an arm cuff whenever possible over a wrist cuff. The arm cuff provides a more accurate measurement of your blood pressure than a wrist cuff does.

4. Stay still and quiet while the measurement is being taken. Talking and moving can mess up the reading.

5. If possible, try to keep your upper arm at the same level as your heart.

6. Place the cuff around the bare skin of your arm and don't inhibit the cuff with any clothing.

Now that you know how to properly take your blood pressure, how do you know if you have high blood pressure or not? You can use the following chart to determine if you have blood pressure in a healthy range:

	Systolic	Diastolic
Normal Blood Pressure	>120	>80
Prehypertension	120-139	80-89
High Stage 1	140-159	90-99
High Stage 2	160+	100+

Note: when you take your blood pressure, you'll see a number like 120/80. The first number (120 in this case) is your systolic blood pressure reading. Your systolic blood pressure is the maximum amount of pressure your heart exerts while beating.

The second number (80 in this example) is your diastolic blood pressure. Your diastolic blood pressure is the measurement of blood pressure in your blood vessels when your heart rests between beats. You would still be considered to have high blood pressure if either reading of your systolic or diastolic blood pressures is high.

Now according to the chart, ideally you want to have a blood pressure reading of less than 120/80. If it's in between the ranges of 120-139/80-89, then you're considered to have elevated blood pressure. You're not considered to have hypertension, but this is something you still need to be cautious of and take the necessary actions to lower it.

If your blood pressure reads between 140-159/90-99, then you're considered to have stage 1 hypertension. If your blood pressure reading measures 160+/100+, then you're considered to have stage 2 hypertension. Stage 2 hypertension is essentially a more serve version of hypertension.

Of course a diagnosis of high blood pressure must be confirmed by a medical professional. If you take a blood pressure reading at home, and you get a high reading, you should see your health care professional for medical guidance and be officially diagnosed with hypertension.

Once you have been officially diagnosed with high blood pressure, what are some things you can do in addition to your doctor's recommendations that can help you lower your blood pressure back down to normal levels?

Tip #1: Stop smoking. If you're currently smoking reducing the amount of cigarettes you smoke or stopping smoking altogether will help you to reduce your blood pressure. The reason for this is because cigarettes contain carbon monoxide. Carbon monoxide decreases your body's ability to carry oxygen, which forces it to have to work harder.

Tip #2: Lose Weight. Carrying around extra weight puts extra strain on your heart. This extra strain in turn forces your heart to have to work harder and thus your blood pressure will increase. The DASH diet will help you to be able to lose weight, which in your will help to decrease your blood pressure.

Tip #3: Limit Alcohol Intake. Drinking excessive amounts of alcohol will increase cortisol levels. Cortisol is a steroid hormone that helps to regulate metabolism and immune response in the body. Research has shown that increased cortisol levels can increase blood pressure (20).

Therefore, by limiting your alcohol intake, you can help to limit unhealthy amounts of cortisol in the body, and thus lower blood pressure. For females, this would mean no more than one alcoholic beverage per day. For males, this would mean no more than 2 alcoholic beverages per day.

And no you can't save it all up and drink it all during the weekend—that's binge drinking! You're still only allowed to have 1-2 drinks per day even on the weekends while on the DASH diet.

Tip #4: Decrease Stress. This may not be the easiest thing to do, but lowering your stress levels can help to decrease your blood pressure. When we are stressed our bodies enter into fight or flight mode. In this state, certain hormones such as adrenaline and cortisol are released to help your body prepare to fight.

Unhealthy amounts of these hormones can increase blood pressure levels. If you're experiencing a lot of stress right now, do what you can to help decrease your stress levels. Practice deep breathing when you notice yourself feeling stressed. Meditate or go for a walk outside. Doing these types of things can help to decrease the amount of stress in your life.

Tip #5: Exercise Regularly. Exercise is a great way to decrease your blood pressure. When you exercise, your blood vessels open up, which allows for more blood flow, and this means that your heart won't have to work as hard thus lowering blood pressure.

Tip #6: Take your medications as prescribed. This tip should be obvious, but it's important to be reminded. Whatever medications you're currently taking, be sure to take them as your doctor has prescribed them to you. Taking the wrong amount of your medications can negatively affect your blood pressure.

Of course following the DASH diet will greatly help you be able to decrease your blood pressure, but these are some additional things you can do to help fight against hypertension.

Health Benefit #3: Weight Loss

Another benefit of the DASH diet (and one I'm sure you're really interested in) is weight loss. Yes, the DASH diet is a great way to help you get back to a healthy bodyweight. The only way your body loses weight is by being in a caloric deficit. A caloric deficit is when your body burns off more calories than you consume.

I'll be going into more specifics about this later on, but for now know that getting in a caloric deficit is critical if you want to lose weight. The DASH diet is a great way to help your body be in a caloric deficit because you're going to be consuming healthier foods such as fruits and vegetables. These types of foods are very nutrient dense, meaning that they contain a lot of vitamins and minerals even though they don't contain a lot of calories.

This is amazing because your body needs certain nutrients in order to feel full and satisfied, which means you'll be able to get full on fewer calories. Imagine when you eat chocolate for example. You can eat a lot of chocolate (which contains a lot of calories) and still not feel full at all.

That won't be the case with the foods you're going to be eating on the DASH diet. Additionally, you'll also be cutting back or completely eliminating certain foods from your diet. Your sugar intake will decrease drastically because you'll only be eating 5 servings of sweets per week. And sugar provides very little if any nutritional value to your body.

You'll also be reducing bad fats such as saturated and trans fat. This'll also help to lower your overall caloric intake because fat contains 9 calories per gram, whereas carbs and protein only contain 4 calories per gram. Even though the DASH diet will be able to help you lose weight, you still must have patience.

The DASH diet isn't like your typical diet fad where you drink a magical formula before bed and lose 10 pounds overnight. No instead, the weight might come off slower than you'd like for it to. You might only lose .5-1 pound per week, but remember this is going to be permanent weight loss. You won't have to worry about gaining this weight back ever again.

Think about how someone gains weight. They usually gain weight slowly and steadily over the years, and then they suddenly realize how much things have gotten out of control. You likely didn't gain all of this weight in a short period of time, so be patient and don't try to lose it all in a short period of time. Remember slow and steady wins the race!

Health Benefit #4: Lower risk of stroke, heart attack, kidney stones, diabetes, and certain types of cancer

When you follow the DASH diet for a long period of time, your chances of developing certain types of diseases is lowered (21). This is great news because health diseases are a big problem in the world right now. Cardiovascular disease is the number one killer in the United States killing over 600,000 Americans each and every year (22).

That's definitely a scary statistic, but there are certainly things within your control that you can do to help lower the risk of developing these diseases. By following the DASH diet, you'll essentially be killing a lot of birds with one stone. The research is sound in showing that when people follow the DASH diet for a significant length of time, their risk for diabetes, certain types of cancer, stroke, and heart attack drops quite a bit (23)(24)(25).

Chapter 5: How to Easily Follow the DASH Diet for a Long Time to Come

When most people start a diet are they successful with it? Sadly no, most people who start a diet, aren't able to stick with it for a very long time, and they're not able to get any noticeable results because of it. If you've ever tried a diet in the past and failed, don't worry, it's not your fault. In most cases, the diet sets you up to fail right from the start.

Luckily the DASH diet isn't like your average diet. It's smart in it's approach to helping you lose weight and get in better health. It's designed in a way to help you be able to sustain the diet for a long time to come. However, even with that being the case, there are some extra things you can do ensure long-term success with the DASH diet eating plan. The following are some good tips and tricks you can use to make sure you get long-term results with this nutrition plan:

Tip #1: Don't Beat Yourself Up

One of the worst things you can do on the DASH diet (or any diet for that matter) is to beat yourself up or feel incredibly guilty whenever you slip up. We're all humans, which means that we're not perfect and we'll make mistakes from time to time. For example, you might eat more ice cream, cake, or another sweet treat than you should of.

What do most people do when they slip up on their diets? They start to feel incredibly guilty, and then since they feel as if their diet is already ruined, they might as well go ahead and eat how they please. This will then of course ruin their nutrition plan indefinitely. Conversely, you must be different from the average person by expecting mistakes to occur when you start the DASH diet plan.

Think about it—if you're going to follow this diet plan for years and years to come, is it really realistic to expect that you'll do everything perfectly and never mess up? Of course it's not! That's why you'll want to set realistic expectations going into the diet.

When you do mess up, take a deep breath and stay calm. Tell yourself it's ok and things like this will happen from time to time. Whenever you fall off track, you can always get back up and keep going. Most people however, feel so ashamed that they decide to give up completely. The only way you will not succeed is if you quit. If you persist and keep going, you'll succeed. Sure there will be some bumps in the road, and it won't be the easiest thing you've ever done, but that's the point!

Anything worth achieving is going to be difficult to achieve. Yes, it might be hard to lose weight and get your blood pressure in check, but the reward will be well worth it. So by planning for and expecting things to not go smoothly 100% of the time, you'll be much more prepared for how you'll need to handle these hic-ups.

Tip #2: Have the Right Mindset Going Into the DASH Diet

Yes the DASH eating plan is technically a "diet," and that's how I've mentioned it throughout this book, but I don't like referring to the DASH eating plan as a diet. When you think of a diet, what do you usually think of? To me when I hear someone say, "I'm going on a diet," I think of something you'll do for the short-term.

You'll go *on* a diet, which means that you'll eventually have to go *off* that same diet. I think of someone who's tired of his or her current health or the way that they look in the mirror. They'll do anything to get some results as quickly as possible. So they'll jump right into an unrealistic diet where they cut out all of the junk food in their diet. Sure they'll get some results at first, but when they can't take it anymore, they'll quit and gain all of the weight back.

And that's the biggest problem with diets. They don't imply long-term, permanent change. They imply putting yourself through a bunch of misery for as long as you can. Then when you can't take it anymore, you give up, and you go back to the way you were eating before you started the diet.

The DASH diet really isn't as much of a diet as it is a lifestyle change. This is how you need to think about the DASH nutrition plan heading into it. If you think about it in terms of a lifestyle change instead of a diet, you'll be much more successful with it. When you think about someone making a lifestyle change, what comes to mind? Probably something positive like lasting changes and thus lasting results.

Now of course does this mean you could take any regular diet, call it a lifestyle change, and poof it's easier to do and you'll be successful with it? No of course not! If a diet is unrealistic from the start, there's no way you'll be able to stick with it for a long time to come. Simply eating nothing but healthy foods such as fruits and vegetables and calling that a lifestyle change instead of a diet is going to have little impact on your results.

The difference with the DASH plan is that it's set up in a way that allows you to actually execute it as a lifestyle change. This is because it allows you to eat up to 5 servings per week of sweets. Doing something like completely eliminating all sweets from your nutrition plan is unrealistic, which is why you'd have to refer to it as a diet.

That's not the case with the DASH eating plan. You're set up from the start to be able to do it for a long time to come, which is far better than most eating plans that fail you before you've even begun.

Tip #3: Actually Eat Your 5 Servings of Sweets per Week

Remember what I just mentioned in the previous step—the DASH plan can be done for a long time to come because it allows you to enjoy your favorite foods from time to time. Even with this being the case, it can still be tempting to want to skip the sweets in an effort to try and obtain even faster results.

I'm telling you right now that you need to avoid that temptation. Eating the sweets (or whatever else you like) is a big part of the eating plan. It'll help to restore your leptin levels, which is an important hormone that regulates how much we eat by telling the brain the amount of fat that's stored in our bodies fat cells.

When we eat sweet treats (such as cake for example) that increases the amount of leptin in our bodies, and this increased leptin will allow us to burn more fat. If we're solely eating low amounts of calories from healthy foods, then our leptin stores will be low, and this will signal to our brains that we need to eat more and hold onto the fat that we currently have stored up.

Not only that, but it's going to give you a break and allow you to reward yourself for eating healthy the rest of the time. Think about it, most people work 5 days and then they have 2 days off, which allows them to relax, recover, and prepare themselves for the following workweek. Imagine if you never got a single day off in your life!

That's essentially what it would be like if you never ate another sweet again in your life. Since this is a lifestyle change, you must be patient. The results will eventually come, and once they do come, you won't have to worry about them going away.

People start to do unrealistic things that won't last when they want fast results. Ironically enough, these people end up achieving no results over a long period of time all because they were chasing something that wasn't going to work from the get-go. Be patient and follow the eating plan exactly as you're supposed to, and you'll have nothing to worry about. And yes that does include eating the 5 servings of sweets per week!

Chapter 6: What Kind of Exercise Works Best with the DASH Diet?

Yes, the DASH diet is a great nutritional plan by itself, but there's another important element we can't forget about—exercise. Of course the DASH diet by itself will certainly be able to provide you with many great health benefits, but these benefits can be maximized with the addition of exercise. The research is clear when it comes to exercise (26). It'll provide the following benefits to you:

- Reduce your risk of cardiovascular disease, stroke, and diabetes
- Make you feel happier
- Reduce feelings of anxiety, depression, and stress
- Help you lose weight
- Help prevent osteoporosis
- Build muscle
- Improve brain health
- Improve sleep quality
- Help you relax
- Increase energy

Yes, you'll notice that many of these benefits of exercise are similar to the pros of the DASH diet. This doesn't mean that you shouldn't exercise because you'll already experience these benefits with your nutrition plan. Instead, this should make you want to exercise more because exercising will amplify these amazing health benefits.

Instead of simply reducing your risk of heart attack and stroke, why not make the risk as low as possible by combining the powers of nutrition with exercise? I get it—most of us are busy people. We have school, work, and a family we have to take care of.

But lack of time is no good excuse for not exercising more. This myth of not having time to workout came about because people think that they have to workout for a long time in order for it to be effective. And you're right, if you had to be in the gym for hours a day, then it'd be reasonable to think that you don't have enough time to workout.

But that isn't the case—you can start to experience some of the benefits of exercise (such as improvement of mood and energizing your body) just by taking a brisk walk for 10 minutes. That equates to less than 1% of your day!

What Type of Exercise Should You Do?

Now that you know the importance of exercise, the real question is what kind of exercise you should be doing. Of course there are many different things that you could be doing and none of them are bad. However, I do think that different things work best for different kinds of people.

At the end of the day, the best kind of exercise for you is the kind of exercise you'll actually do. You might like cardio more than weightlifting or vice-versa and that's ok. Ideally you would do both because there are certain benefits you can only get from doing cardio, and there are certain benefits you can get from weightlifting. With that being said, let's get into some specifics for what you should be doing in terms of exercise:

Weightlifting

Many times when people think of lifting weights, they think of macho bodybuilders. You don't have to have the end goal of looking like a bodybuilder if you want to lift weights. And no, lifting weights won't make you look like a bodybuilder. Resistance training has been shown to increase bone density, which can help to prevent osteoporosis when you're older (27).

Weightlifting is also great for building and maintaining muscle mass. You may or may not be interested in building muscle mass, but it'll decrease as you age. This decrease in muscle mass can lead to disability and injury. The cool thing is that you don't have to workout 5-6 times a week to start seeing these benefits.

Studies have shown that you only need to engage in resistance training 2-3 times per week to start reaping the rewards (28). Of course, you may not be sure what to do when you're at the gym but fear not. The following is a good workout you can do as a beginner to lifting weights:

- Back Squats 3 sets of 10 reps 90 seconds rest between sets
- Dumbbell Military Press 3 sets of 10 reps 60 seconds rest between sets
- Lat Pulldown 3 sets of 12 reps 60 seconds rest between sets
- Incline Dumbbell Bench Press 3 sets of 8 reps 90 seconds rest between sets
- Standing Dumbbell Curls 3 sets of 10 reps 60 seconds rest between sets
- Tricep Rope Pushdowns 3 sets of 12 reps 60 seconds rest between sets
- Planks 3 sets of holding the plank position for as long as you can

Side Note #1: A set is a group of consecutive repetitions. A repetition is one complete motion of an exercise. And the rest period is how long of a break you'll take until you start the next set.

For example, let's say you're completing 3 sets of 10 reps and resting 90 seconds in between sets for the barbell squat exercise. You'll squat down and stand back up, completing the movement of the exercise and one rep. You'll repeat that motion 9 more times for a total of 10 repetitions. That will complete the set and you will begin your rest period.

Once your 90-second rest period is up, you'll start the next set and perform another 10 repetitions. That will complete set number 2, and you'll rest another 90 seconds. Once that time period is up, you'll complete the final set of 10 repetitions, and then you'll move onto the next exercise.

Side Note #2: Lift as much weight as you possibly can for the given rep range. Initially, you won't know how much weight to use so you'll have to take your best guess. For example, let's say you're doing bench press for 8 reps. You think you can lift around 150 pounds for that many reps, but on your first set, you easily complete 10 reps.

This means the weight is too light and you need to increase it for the next set. On the next set, you lift 165 pounds and struggle to complete the 8th rep. This is what you want to happen and it means you've found a good weight to use. Once you can complete all 3 sets of 8 reps with 165 pounds, move up to 170 the next time you bench press. If you can't complete 8 reps for all 3 sets, stick with 165 until you can. Here's an example:

Workout 1: Bench Press with 165 pounds
Set 1: 8 reps
Set 2: 8 reps
Set 3: 7 reps

Because you only completed 7 reps on the last set, stick with 165 for the next workout—

Workout 2: Bench Press with 165 pounds
Set 1: 8 reps
Set 2: 8 reps
Set 3: 8 reps

Because you completed all 3 sets of 8 reps, move up to 170 on your next workout with bench press.

It's better to use a weight that's too heavy and miss a rep or two than it is to use a weight that's too light and leave some reps in the tank. For example, it's better to do 170 pounds and only complete 6 reps instead of 8 opposed to using 155 pounds and stopping at 8 reps even though you could've easily done more reps.

Side Note #3: You can set up your gym schedule however you like based on the number of days you're going to be working out. The specific days of the week you workout versus when you rest isn't important.

For example, if you're going to workout 2 times per week you could workout on Tuesday and Friday or Wednesday and Saturday for example. The main thing you'll want to do when working out 2 days per week is have at least 48 hours of rest in between the workouts.

If you're going to workout 3 times per week you could workout on Monday, Wednesday, and Friday. You could also workout on Tuesday, Thursday, and Saturday. Choose whatever works best for you and your schedule. The main thing when you're working out three days per week is to make sure that you're taking at least one day of rest in between your workouts.

Playing Sports

If the idea of running on a treadmill sounds boring to you, then doing something such as playing sports can be a good option for you. Sports are essentially an intense form of cardio disguised in the form of a game.

It doesn't matter what makes you do cardio as long as you do it, and sports are a great way to break up the monotony of doing cardio on a machine. Interestingly enough, playing high-impact sports such as basketball or soccer have been shown to increase bone density more so than non-impact sports such as swimming (29).

Running

Aside from playing sports, you can also go the more traditional route of cardio and do regular running such as jogging or sprinting. You can do long steady-state cardio where you run at the same pace for a certain length of time, or you can do a more intense version of cardio such as high-intensity interval training.

Either form of cardio will provide you with positive health effects. Doing steady-state cardio is simple and doesn't need much explaining—you run at the same pace for a predetermined length of time or distance.

High-intensity interval training (HIIT for short) can be a little bit harder to grasp if you've never heard of it before. HIIT is simply alternating between high-intensity cardio and low intensity cardio. It can be performed by running outside, or on any cardio machine of your choosing at the gym. Here's an example of a HIIT workout you could do on a treadmill:

-Run at 7.5 mph for 1 minute
-Walk at 3.5 mph for 1 minute

Now of course if you need to adjust the intensity of the HIIT then you can certainly do so. You can alter the run-walk ratios (i.e. run for 30 seconds and walk for 1.5 minutes), or you can decrease the intensity of each run (i.e. run at 6 mph instead of 7.5). And if what I prescribed is too easy, then ramp up the intensity accordingly.

Walking

Walking tends to get a bad reputation. People think that it's only something unfit people do. I used to fall into this line of thinking as well and it couldn't be any further from the truth. In fact, there are certain health benefits that you'll get from walking that you can't get from the more intense forms of cardio. For starters, walking is a low-impact form of exercise.

This means that it won't be as strenuous on your bones, tendons, and ligaments as other forms of exercise might be. It's also incredibly simple to do. You don't have to worry about changing into gym clothes and driving to the gym if you don't want to. You can walk just about anywhere whenever you feel like it.

Finally walking helps to cleanse the lymphatic system. While the circulatory system relies on the heart to move blood, the lymphatic system doesn't have a pump like the heart does to keep it going. It instead relies on bodily movement to keep on going.

The lymphatic system is important for ridding the body of toxins, waste, and other unwanted materials. And engaging the lymphatic system is simple; all it really takes is 10-20 minutes of brisk walking per day. This'll be a great start to get the lymphatic system moving and start clearing your body of harmful toxins.

Chapter 7: Setting Up and Starting Your DASH Diet Plan

So far, you've learned a lot of information about the DASH eating plan and what it can do for you. However, putting all of the info together into an actionable plan can be a little confusing and difficult.

In this chapter, I'm going to give you the step-by-step process to set-up your DASH diet nutrition plan so that you can get started with it as soon as possible. Let's dive right in...

Step #1: Don't Forget About Calorie Quantity!

When it comes to calories, many people only regard the quality of the calories as important. For example, an avocado would be considered healthier and therefore better than a candy bar. Yes, the avocado will provide your body with way more vitamins and nutrients than the candy bar ever will. However, depending on the amounts, the avocado will likely contain more calories overall than the candy bar.

This is why you must also take into consideration the quantity of the foods you're eating as well. Many people don't think that it's possible to overeat healthy foods, but it certainly is possible. For example, you could eat the following meal for breakfast:

- 1 cup of oatmeal (300 calories)
- 1 cup of 1% milk (103 calories)

- Handful of blueberries (30 calories)
- 1 tbsp. of almond butter (100 calories)
- 1 slice of toast (75 calories)
- Total calories: 608

608 total calories is quite a lot. Of course, this meal would be very filling and nutritious, but it's still more than most would expect when added up. This is important to know because it's a myth that simply starting a healthy diet, such as the DASH diet, will guarantee weight loss when, in fact, it doesn't.

You must be able to track your calories and understand how your body works in regards to weight loss and weight gain, and it all comes down to energy balance. Every day your body needs the energy to breathe, digest food, regulate body temperature, allow your organs to function, etc. We give our body the energy it needs to perform these functions through the foods that we eat also known as calories.

When we eat more calories than our bodies need (caloric surplus), we'll store some of the calories as fat so we can use them later. When we eat exactly the amount of calories our body needs (maintenance), we'll neither gain nor lose weight. And finally, when we eat fewer calories than our body needs (caloric deficit), we'll use some of our stored fat for energy. Here's an example:

Let's pretend that Craig's maintenance calories are 2,300 (don't worry, we'll figure this out in the next step).

- If Craig eats more than 2,300 calories, he'll be in a caloric surplus and will start to gain weight.
- If Craig eats right at 2,300 calories, he'll be eating at his maintenance levels and will neither gain nor lose weight.
- If Craig eats less than 2,300 calories, he'll be in a caloric deficit and will start losing weight.

So if Craig wants to start losing weight, he knows he must eat less than 2,300 calories per day. That's a great start that most people will never even consider. The next thing he must determine is what he eats because it does matter. The point isn't to eat whatever you want as long as you're in a deficit. The point is to plan ahead so you know the direction you're heading in and to eat high-quality foods to feel great and get healthy.

For example, let's say you eat 150 calories worth of fruit and vegetables, and I eat 150 calories from a chocolate bar. Are we equal? Well kinda. The total amount of calories we ate was the same.

There's no arguing this because a calorie *is* a calorie, just like a yard of wood is the same length as a yard of sheet metal. However, the quality of the calories is vastly different. The fruits and vegetables you ate will provide you with fiber, keeping you fuller for a longer period of time. The fruits and vegetables also contain way more vitamins and minerals than the chocolate bar does.

And when you're eating fewer calories overall to lose weight, it's important that you make those calories count. You want to be consuming high-quality foods because that's how you'll stay full for long periods of time even when your calories are being restricted. Now let's move on and determine how many calories you should be eating...

Step #2: Determine Your Resting Metabolic Rate

Like I mentioned in the previous step, your body needs energy (calories) in order to continue on with all of its chemical functions like breathing, digesting food, organ function, etc. The amount of calories you burn on any given day is your resting metabolic rate (rmr). Once you figure out your body's rmr, you can then determine how many calories you need to eat to start burning fat.

Determining your rmr is simple—multiply your bodyweight in pounds by 13.
Let's use myself as an example:

Bodyweight=205 pounds
205 x 13= RMR of 2,665

This means that if I eat less than 2,665 calories, I'll be in a caloric deficit and will start to lose weight. If I eat more than 2,665 calories, I'll be in a caloric surplus and will start to gain weight. And finally, if I eat exactly 2,665 calories, I'll be at maintenance and will neither gain nor lose weight.

The question is—how big of a caloric deficit do you need to create in order for it to translate into pounds lost? There are about 3,500 calories in one pound of fat (30), meaning that you must create a cumulative caloric deficit of 3,500 calories in order to lose 1 pound. So if you divide 3,500 by 7 days in a week, you'll need to create an average daily caloric deficit of 500 calories to lose 1 pound per week.

Referring back to the example from above, here's what that would translate to:

RMR- 2,665 − 500= 2,165

This means that I need to eat 2,165 calories every day if I want to lose 1 pound per week. The more weight you have to lose, the larger the caloric deficit you can create. For example, you could eat at a caloric deficit of 750 calories and lose 1.5 pounds per week, or you could eat at a deficit of 1,000 calories to lose 2 pounds per week.

Essentially, for every 250 calories you can expect to lose an additional .5-pound. The key is to not get carried away. You might want to lose all of the weight as soon as possible and jump right into a 1,000-calorie caloric deficit.

That may not be the best idea. For most people, losing 1 pound per week by creating a 500-calorie caloric deficit is golden. Imagine yourself a year from now being 52 pounds lighter without having to put forth much effort! That's much better than spinning your wheels trying to lose 100 pounds in that same time frame.

Of course you may not be doing the DASH diet to lose weight, and it's okay if that's the case for you. If you're following the DASH eating plan to get some of the health benefits out of it, then you certainly don't have to be nearly as strict in regards to how many calories you're eating.

You'll still want to eat the right foods of course, but you won't have to be as strict with keeping track of your calories. Of course you still can if you want to, just to make sure you stay on track with maintaining your bodyweight. For example, let's say you determined your resting metabolic rate was 2,000 calories. You could still measure out and eat 2,000 calories a day to ensure that you won't gain any unwanted weight.

Step #3: Determine Serving Sizes

Now that you know how many calories it is that you need to be eating, all you need to do from here is start eating according to the DASH diet plan. In an earlier chapter, I went over the number of servings you need to eat per day for each food group. Before I get into how to adjust serving sizes based on your caloric needs, how can you tell how much a serving size is?

Serving sizes will vary depending on the type of food that you're eating. For example, one serving of raw broccoli is ½ cup. On the other hand, 1 cup of milk is a serving of dairy.

Unfortunately, it's not as easy as saying one cup of anything equals one serving size.

The best thing you can do is read the nutritional label of the foods you're eating to see what the measured serving sizes are. Sometimes you'll have to eyeball the amount of food you're eating and that's okay. Here's a chart to give you some accurate measurements when you have to eyeball the amount of food you're eating:

Item	Approximate Equivalency
Baseball	~1 cup
Small Computer Mouse	~1/2 cup
Deck of Cards	~3 ounces of meat
Golf Ball	~1 ounce/2 tbsp.
CD	~1 ounce of sliced meat
Nine-Volt Battery	~1 ounce of cheese

In addition to using the eyeball test, you can also buy a food scale. A food scale will be able to tell you how many grams are in a certain food item, which you can then use to determine the serving size. Now, in the earlier chapter, the following serving sizes were recommended for each of these different food groups:

- Vegetables: 4-5 servings per day
- Fruit: 4-5 servings per day
- Nuts, Seeds, and Dried Beans: 3 servings per week
- Dairy: 2-3 servings per day
- Meats, Poultry, and Fish: 1-2 servings per day
- Fats and Oils: 2 per day
- Whole Grains: 6-8 per day
- Sweets: 5 per week

These recommendations are based on a standard 2,000 calorie a day diet. In fact, everywhere you look, food labels and percentages are based on a 2,000 calorie a day diet. The reason why it was set up this way was to because the FDA needed benchmarks for average calorie consumption and 2,000 was the number they came up with.

They knew that people have varying caloric needs, but putting different daily percentage values for a wide range of caloric intakes would take up way too much space. 2,000 is also a very easy number to work with if you need to convert certain values to meet your needs.

So if from the previous steps, you determined that you need to eat 1,600 calories per day, does this mean that you should eat the serving size recommendations for a 2,000 calorie diet? Definitely not! You'll want to make sure that you adjust the serving sizes accordingly to fit your specific needs. Here are a couple of different charts you can use to help you determine your serving sizes based on your caloric needs.

Serving Sizes based on a 1,600 calorie per day diet:

- Vegetables: 3-4 per day
- Fruits: 3-4 per day
- Nuts, Seeds, and Dried Beans: 2 per week
- Dairy: 2 per day
- Meats, Poultry, and Fish: 1 per day
- Fats and Oils: 1-2 per day
- Whole Grains: 6 per day
- Sweets: 3-4 per week

Serving Sizes based on a 3,000 calorie per day diet:

- Vegetables: 6 per day
- Fruits: 6 per day
- Nuts, Seeds, and Dried Beans: 1 per day
- Dairy: 3-4 per day
- Meats, Poultry, and Fish: 2-3 per day
- Fats and Oils: 3-4 per day
- Whole Grains: 10-12 per day
- Sweets: 6-7 per week

These charts will help to cover a wider range of caloric needs, but what if you need to eat 1,800 calories per day for example? In that case, go in between the 2,000 and 1,600 calorie per day plan to figure out approximately how many servings you need to be eating per day.

For example, on the 1,600 calorie plan, you'll be eating 6 servings of whole grains per day. On the 2,000 calorie diet plan, you'll be eating 6-8 servings of whole grains per day. Therefore, if you needed to eat 1,800 calories per day, you could eat 7 servings of whole grains per day.

The 1,600 calorie plan also calls for 3-4 servings of vegetables per day, and the 2,000 calorie diet plan calls for 4-5 servings of vegetables per day. If you're eating 1,800 calories per day, you should therefore eat 4 servings of vegetables per day.

The main goal with servings isn't to get it down exactly right, but to give you a good estimate of how much you should be eating of certain food groups. If you're eating 1,800 calories per day, and you eat 5 servings of vegetables one day, don't sweat it. The main point is to give you an estimation of how you should be eating.

Step #4: Execute on the DASH Eating Plan

Congratulations, by this point you've completed most of the hard work in setting up your nutrition plan! All you need to do is follow through. You know how many calories it is that you should be eating per day, and you also know how much of each food group you should be eating.

All you have to do from here is execute and start getting results! Of course, this isn't the last step in the process because things don't always go exactly the way they're planned out. Sometimes we have to make adjustments along the way...

Step #5: Make Necessary Adjustments

In order to know that you're getting all of the numbers to line up accordingly, you'll need to track how many calories it is that you're eating. Remember, what gets measured gets managed. The best way to be able to do this is to download a calorie counting app on your smartphone. All you have to do is type in the foods that you ate, and in what amounts, and the app will track the how many calories you've eaten for the day.

This is an extremely easy way to make sure that you're on track to hit your caloric goals as well as your serving sizes for the different food groups. Of course, you don't have to use a calorie counting app if you don't want to. You can use a pen and paper if you're old school. It might be a little bit more tedious, but it's still effective.

Simply measure out how many calories are in the foods you're eating by looking at the food label or weighing it on a food scale. From there, you'll simply write down what foods you ate and the total number of calories it contained. Then at the end of the day, you can add up your totals to see where you stand.

Yes, calorie counting is tedious, but there's no other way you're going to be able to fully know if you're on the right track or not. By measuring your calories, you'll be able to know exactly where you stand, and you'll be able to make any necessary adjustments. For example, let's say you need to eat 2,000 calories a day on the DASH diet.

Unless you track what you're eating, how do you really know that you're eating 2,000 calories a day? You simply don't! Once you start tracking your calories, you might realize that you've been eating 2,300 calories per day instead of 2,000— whoops!

That's why it's critical that you measure and track how much food it is that you're eating. After a while, you'll get a good feel for how much it is that you need to eat per day. At that point, you can start to eyeball things more and be less strict with measuring your calories. Until you reach that point though, track your calories!

Ultimately, the point of all of these steps is to teach you how to be self-sufficient with the DASH diet plan. Remember the old saying, if you give a man a fish, you feed him for a day. If you teach a man how to fish, you feed him for a lifetime. Sure I could simply tell you to eat these certain foods and start getting results, but I know that won't last.

In order to get lasting results, you need to be adaptable and make certain adjustments when necessary. Your caloric needs won't always stay the same for example, or you might need to change up serving size for a certain food group. If I simply told you what to do and then ran away, you'd be left clueless as to what to do. Instead my goal is to not just give you the necessary tools you need to be successful with the DASH diet, but also teach you how to use those tools.

That's why following this last step of the process is so important. If you don't measure your weight, you won't know how many calories you need to eat. If you don't know how many calories you need to eat, then you won't know the proper serving sizes for each food group.

And finally, if you don't measure and track what you're eating, then you won't know if you're eating the proper amounts of each food group. It all comes down to preparation. When you fail to prepare, you prepare to fail!

Chapter 8: 14-Day DASH Diet Sample Meal Plan

The following is a 14-day sample meal plan you can use to give you an idea of how you should be eating while on the DASH diet plan. This is simply meant to help guide you and ease you into starting the nutrition plan. It's not to be used as a crutch.

Recall the phrase, "if you give a man a fish, you feed him for a day. If you teach a man to fish, you feed him for life." It wouldn't be practical for me to tell you exactly how to eat each and every day. If I tried to do that, you would end up failing.

You wouldn't be able to adapt to different situations you'd find yourself in. For example, let's say you're at an office party, and you're not able to eat exactly what the meal plan laid out for you. What do you do? You'd likely freeze up and paralyze yourself because you don't know how to adapt yourself to the given situation.

On the other hand, if you know all of the ins and outs of the DASH diet (which you should by now), then you'll know what you are and aren't allowed to eat at the office party. You'll still be able to enjoy yourself without having to constantly worry if you broke your diet plan or not. With that being said, this sample meal plan is based on a 2,000 calorie a day diet. Be sure to adjust the serving and portion sizes accordingly to fit your caloric needs.

Note: You can break up these meal plan ideas into smaller meals with snacks if you like. I made the meal plans with just breakfast, lunch, and dinner, but you can modify it to have snacks if that's how you like to eat.

For example, let's say for breakfast you're going to eat 1 cup of oatmeal, 1 cup of skim milk, ½ cup of raspberries, and 1 medium banana. You could skip out on eating the banana as part of your breakfast and instead eat it a couple of hours later as a snack. It can be done either way because it works out to the same amount of calories in the end. Choose whatever works best for you and how it is that you prefer to eat.

Additionally, replace certain foods as necessary. For example, if a meal calls for ½ cup of blueberries and you like raspberries more, then go ahead and eat ½ cup of raspberries instead of blueberries. Or if you like cauliflower more than carrots, then go ahead and replace the carrots with cauliflower.

Yes, variety is good, but don't feel like you have to eat a certain fruit or vegetable that you hate when you could easily replace it with something else. Do what works best for you and will allow you to stick to this diet for a long time to come.

Finally, I didn't include any of the sweets in the meal plan. Feel free to add in whatever sweets you like throughout the week up to your allotted number of servings.

Day 1:

Breakfast

- 2 Slices of Whole Wheat Toast
- 2 Tablespoons of Natural Peanut Butter (one tbsp. per slice of toast)
- 1 Medium Apple
- ½ Cup of Your Choice of Berries

Lunch

- 3 Ounces of Lean Turkey
- 1 Cup of Broccoli
- 1 Cup of Quinoa
- 1.5 Ounces of Low-Fat Yogurt

Dinner

- 3 ounces of grilled chicken
- ½ Cup of Steamed Cauliflower
- ½ Cup of Steamed Bell Peppers
- 1 Cup of Brown Rice
- 1 Medium Orange

Day 2:

Breakfast:

- 2 Scrambled Eggs
- ½ of a Whole-Wheat Pita Pocket
- ½ of a Medium Grapefruit

Lunch:

- 3 Ounces of Cod
- 2 Teaspoons of Olive Oil
- ½ Cup of Mixed Berries
- 1 Cup of Steamed Broccoli
- 1 Whole-Wheat Roll

Dinner:

- 2 Cups of Whole-Wheat Spaghetti Noodles
- ½ Cup of Grated Parmesan Cheese
- ½ Cup of Tomato Sauce
- 2 Ounces of Lean Beef

Day 3:

Breakfast:

- 1 Cup of Oatmeal
- ½ Cup of Raspberries
- 1 Cup of Skim Milk
- 1 Medium Banana

Lunch:

Salad Consisting of the Following:

- 3 Ounces of Lean Grilled Chicken
- 3 Cups of Leafy Green Vegetables
- ½ Cup of Cumcumber
- ½ Tablespoon of Flax Seeds

On the Side:

- ½ Slice of Toast

Dinner:

- 1 Cup of Roasted Potatoes
- 3 Ounces of Roast Beef
- ½ Cup of Roasted Carrots
- ½ Cup of Roasted Onions

Day 4:

Breakfast:

- 3 Hard Boiled Eggs
- 2 Slices of Turkey Bacon
- 6 Ounces of Freshly Squeezed Orange Juice
- 6 Ounces of Low-Fat Yogurt

Lunch:

Sandwich Consisting of the Following:

- 2 Slices of Whole-Wheat Bread
- 3 Ounces of Packaged Tuna
- 1 Tablespoon of Mayonnaise

On the Side:

- ½ Cup of Kale
- ½ Cup of Tomatoes
- ½ Cup of Spinach
- ½ Cup of Pineapple

Dinner:

- 3 Ounces of Lean Venison
- 1 Cup of Sweet Potatoes
- ½ Cup of Roasted Carrots
- ½ Cup of Roasted Bell Pepper

Day 5:

Breakfast:

Breakfast Sandwich Consisting of the Following:

- 2 Slices of Whole Wheat Toast
- 3 Slices of Turkey Bacon
- 1 Fried Egg

On the side:

- 1 Medium Apple

Lunch:

Turkey Roll-Ups Consisting of:

- 3 Ounces of Lean Turkey Meat
- 1/4 Cup of Cheese
- 2-3 Large Leaves of Romaine Lettuce
- 2 Teaspoons of Mustard

On the Side:

- 1 Medium Apple
- ½ Cup of Mixed Broccoli and Cauliflower

Dinner:

Stuffed Bell Pepper Consisting of:

- 1 Full-Sized Bell Pepper
- 1/4 Cup of Low-Fat Cheese
- ½ Cup of Chickpeas
- ¼ Cup of Dried Apricots

Day 6:

Breakfast:

- 1 Cup of Oat Bran
- 1 Cup of Skim Milk
- ½ Cup of Mixed Berries
- 6 Ounces of Freshly Squeezed Pineapple Juice

Lunch:

Sandwich Consisting of the following:

- 2 Slices of Whole-Wheat Bread
- 3 Ounces of Lean Turkey
- ¼ Cup of Low-Fat Cheese
- 2 Teaspoons of Mustard

On the side:

- 1/3 Cup of Almonds
- 1 Medium Banana
- ½ Cup of Your Choice of Vegetables

Dinner:

Fish Tacos Consisting of:

- 3 Ounces of Tilapia
- 2 Whole-Wheat Tortillas
- 1/4 Cup of Low-Fat Cheese

On the side:

- 1 Medium Peach
- 1 Cup of Mixed Vegetables

Day 7:

Breakfast:

- 1 Whole-Wheat Bagel
- 2 Tablespoons of Natural Almond or Peanut Butter
- 1 Medium Pear
- 1 Cup of Skim Milk

Lunch:

Salad Consisting of the following:

- 4 Cups of Spring Mix Salad
- ¼ Cup of Severed Almonds
- ½ Cup of Orange Slices
- 2 Tablespoons of Low-Fat Dressing

Dinner:

- 3 Ounces of Salmon
- 1 Cup of Strawberries
- 1 Cup of Asparagus
- 1 Small Biscuit
- 2 Teaspoons of Olive Oil

Day 8:

Breakfast:

- 1 Cup of Oatmeal
- 1 Cup of Skim Milk
- ½ Cup of Strawberries
- ½ Cup of Mango

Lunch:

Baked Potato Consisting of the Following:

- 1 Large Potato
- ¼ Cup of Shredded Cheese
- ¼ Cup of Bacon Bits
- 1 Tablespoon of Reduced Fat Sour Cream

On the side:

- 1 cup of mixed broccoli, cauliflower, and bell pepper

Dinner:

- 3 Ounces of Lean Steak
- 1 Cup of Brown Rice
- 1 Teaspoon of Olive Oil
- ½ Cup of Steamed Asparagus and Carrots

Day 9:

Breakfast:

- 2 Slices of Whole-Wheat Toast
- 2 Tablespoons of Natural Almond Butter
- 1 Medium Peach
- 1 Cup of Skim Milk

Lunch:

Salad Consisting of the Following:

- 3 Ounces of Lean Chicken
- 2 Cups of Spring Mix Salad
- 2 Tablespoons of Low-Fat Dressing
- ½ Cup of Raspberries
- 1.5 Ounces of Low-Fat Cheese

Dinner:

Stir Fry Consisting of the Following:

- 2 Cups of Snow Peas
- ½ Cup of Kale
- 2 Tablespoons of Olive Oil
- 2 Cups of Quinoa
- ½ Cup of Mixed Nuts

Day 10:

Breakfast:

- 3 Scrambled Eggs
- 1 Slice of Whole-Wheat Toast
- 2 Slices of Turkey Bacon
- 6 Ounces of Yogurt
- 6 Ounces of Freshly Squeezed Orange Juice

Lunch:

Turkey and Swiss Sandwich Consisting of the Following:

- 3 Ounces of Lean Turkey
- 2 Teaspoons of Mayonnaise
- 2 Slices of a Tomato
- 1 Slice of Swiss Cheese
- 2 Slices of Whole-Wheat Bread

On the side:

½ Cup of Cauliflower and Broccoli

Dinner:

- 2 Cups of Whole-Wheat Angel Pasta
- ½ Cup of Grated Parmesan Cheese
- ½ Cup of Tomato Sauce
- 2 Ounces of Lean Venison
- 1 Cup of Mixed Vegetables

Day 11:

Breakfast:

- 1 Cup of Bran Flakes Cereal
- 1 Cup of Skim Milk
- 1 Medium Apple
- 1 Slice of Whole-Wheat Toast

Lunch:

Turkey Roll-Ups Consisting of:

- 3 Ounces of Lean Turkey Meat
- 1/4 Cup of Cheddar Cheese
- 2-3 Large Leaves of Romaine Lettuce
- 2 Teaspoons of Mustard

On the Side:

- 1 Medium Pear
- ½ Cup of Mixed Brussell Sprouts

Dinner:

Fish Tacos Consisting of:

- 3 Ounces of Cod
- 2 Whole-Wheat Tortillas
- 1/4 Cup of Low-Fat Cheese

On the side:

- ½ of a Medium Grapefruit
- 1 Cup of Mixed Vegetables

Day 12:

Breakfast:

- 1 Cup of Oat Bran
- 1 Cup of Skim Milk
- 1 Medium Orange
- 1 Slice of Whole Wheat Toast
- 1 Tablespoon of Natural Peanut Butter

Lunch:

Salad Consisting of the Following:

- 1 Boiled Egg
- 3 Ounces of Packaged Tuna
- 2 Cups of Leafy Green Vegetables
- ½ Cup of Diced Tomatoes
- 2 Tablespoons of Low-Fat Dressing

Dinner:

Hamburger consisting of the following:

- 3 Ounces of Lean Beef
- 1 Whole-Wheat Bun
- 1 Leaf of Romaine Lettuce
- 1 Slice of a Tomato
- 1 Slice of Cheese
- 2 Teaspoons of Mustard

On the Side:

- 1 Cup of Mixed Vegetables

Day 13:

Breakfast:

Sandwich Consisting of:

- 1 Cooked Egg
- 2 Slices of Turkey Bacon
- 2 Slices of Whole Wheat Toast
- 2 Teaspoons of Mustard
- 1 Slice of Cheese

On the side:

- 1 Medium Banana

Lunch:

Salad Consisting of the following:

- 4 Cups of Spring Mix Salad
- ¼ Cup of Severed Almonds
- ½ Cup of Raspberries
- 2 Tablespoons of Low-Fat Dressing

On the side:

- 1 Whole-Wheat Roll

Dinner:

- 1 Cup of Roasted Sweet Potatoes
- 3 Ounces of Roast Beef
- ½ Cup of Roasted Bell Peppers
- ½ Cup of Roasted Onions

Day 14:

Breakfast:

- 1 Whole-Wheat Bagel
- 2 Tablespoons of Natural Almond or Peanut Butter
- 6 Ounces of Yogurt
- ½ Medium Grapefruit

Lunch:

Sandwich Consisting of:

- 3 Ounces of Lean Chicken Breast
- 2 Slices of Whole Wheat Bread
- 1 Slice of Pepper Jack Cheese
- 1 Slice of a Tomato
- 2 Teaspoons of Mayonnaise

On the Side:

- ½ Cup of Cantaloupe
- ½ Cup of Your Choice of Vegetables

Dinner:

- 3 Ounces of Salmon
- 1 Cup of Brown Rice
- 1 Cup of Cooked Spinach
- 1 Tablespoon of Mixed Nuts
- 1 Whole-Wheat Biscuit

Chapter 9: Frequently Asked Questions

How many meals should I eat per day?

You can eat as many meals as you like throughout the day. Meal frequency doesn't matter for weight loss (31), but the total amount of calories you eat does. So eat however is easiest for you and your schedule.

I myself prefer to eat 3 meals a day and that works great for most people. However, feel free to eat 6 times per day or even as little as once per day. As long as you're hitting your servings for each food group and the correct number of calories you'll be fine.

How Spot On Do I Have to Be With My Serving Sizes?

The serving sizes are there to give you a good idea of how much of certain food groups you should be eating. You don't have to be spot on with each and every food group each and every day—that would drive just about anybody nuts. There might be one day for example where you eat an extra two servings of dairy.

If that's the case, then over the next 2 days you could eat 1 less serving of dairy to balance it out. You're not always going to be perfect with it, and that's ok! What matters is that you stay within a serving or so of what's being recommended and you'll be fine.

How much water should I drink on a daily basis?

Your body is made up of about 60% water, so it's important to consume water for several reasons:

>Helps keep your joints and ligaments fluid, which can help prevent injury
>Helps control your caloric intake
>Flushes out toxins
>Improves skin quality
>Improves kidney function
>Improves your focus

Many people recommend that you should drink 1 gallon of water per day. This is a blanket answer that doesn't meet individual needs. This recommendation would have a 100-pound woman drinking the same amount of water as a 200-pound man. Absurd!

Other health experts advise drinking eight 8-ounce glasses (64 ounces total) of water a day. But again 64 ounces isn't going to be enough for most people. What should you do then? I don't keep track of my water intake—I go by how I feel and the color of my urine.

Your body's own thirst mechanism will be accurate in telling you if you need more water. If you feel thirsty, go drink some water. If not, you're probably ok. You can also use the color of your urine to judge how hydrated you are. If your urine is yellow, then you should drink more water. If it's clear, then you should be good to go. This keeps things simple and it's one less thing you have to keep track of.

How Fast Should I Lose Weight?

The more weight you have to lose, the faster the rate at which you can lose the weight. For example, if you have 50+

pounds to lose, you can lose weight at a rate of 2 pounds or more per week. If you only have 5 pounds to lose, then you'll lose weight at a rate of .5 pound per week.

For most people, losing 1 pound per week is the sweet spot. You'll be creating an average caloric deficit of 500 calories daily. At this pace, you'll be losing weight fairly quickly and you won't be miserable all of the time from a complete lack of calories.

What do I do once I reach my goal bodyweight?

Contrary to what you might be thinking, things aren't going to be that much different from what you've been doing to lose weight. You still need to follow the DASH diet and continue eating in the same manner that you previously were. This means that you should still keep the same eating schedule and keep eating similar meals to the ones that you were eating to lose weight.

However, there's one difference between maintenance and creating a caloric deficit to lose weight. The difference is that you get to consume more calories! How many calories? Well, this is pretty easy to figure out as a matter of fact.

Step #1: Determine at what rate you were losing weight (i.e. 1 pound per week)

Step #2: Translate pounds lost per week into calories
    .5-pound lost per week= 250 calories
    1 pound lost per week= 500 calories
    1.5 pounds lost per week= 750 calories
    2 pounds lost per week= 1,000 calories, etc.

Step #3: Add in those additional calories to what you were previously eating to maintain your new weight.

For example, let's say someone was losing weight at a rate of 1 pound per week by eating 1,850 calories per day. Once he hits his goal weight, he needs to eat 2,350 calories (1,850+500) per day to maintain his new weight.

What if I hit a plateau and I stop losing weight at my regular pace?

Let's say you been losing weight just fine, but then all of the sudden you hit a wall and stop losing weight. In this case, take your new current bodyweight (which should be a lower number from when you first started) and multiply that by 13.

Take that number and subtract 250 from it. This will be your new daily caloric intake for you to lose weight.

This will have you losing weight at a rate of approximately .5-pound per week. You may have previously been losing weight at a rate of 1-pound per week, but now you'll lose at a rate of .5-pound per week.

This is because I don't want you to drastically reduce your calories all of the sudden and because if you've hit a plateau you're likely very close to hitting your goal weight anyway.

What if I'm not losing or gaining weight eating 13 calories per pound of bodyweight?

If you've been struggling to lose weight eating 13 calories per pound of bodyweight, then I recommend using a different method to set your calories. Before I get into that though, you must first make sure you were actually eating 13 calories per pound of bodyweight minus 500 calories to lose 1 pound per week. It's easy to overestimate the amount of calories you're eating, and this could be the reason why you're not seeing results.

Once you've made sure you've accurately been tracking your calories, you can take your goal bodyweight, multiply it by 11, and then eat that many calories (don't subtract anything from the final calculated number).

Yes, I understand that your goal bodyweight will be a random number that you think you'll look good at, so take your best guess. Start on the higher side and work your way down from there if you still aren't losing weight.

Here's an example for a 250-pound male.

Current Weight 250

Goal Bodyweight 200

200x11= 2,200 daily calories

Let's say once this person reaches his goal of 200 pounds he's still not satisfied with how he looks. From there he can simply set a new goal bodyweight (i.e. 190 pounds for example) and go from there.

Conclusion:

You now know everything about the DASH diet that you need to in order to be successful with it. It's been voted the best diet as many times as it has for good reason. You can certainly get great results with it, and now it's up to you. If you stay dedicated and follow the plan as it is, you'll start to see results. It won't always be easy, but as long as you don't give up, you'll get there in the end! Finally if you have any questions I'd be happy to answer them! You can reach me by emailing me at thomas@rohmerfitness.com Thanks!

Sources

(1) https://www.cdc.gov/bloodpressure/faqs.htm

(2) https://www.cdc.gov/bloodpressure/index.htm

(3) http://www.collective-evolution.com/2017/02/27/shocking-fast-food-statistics-how-you-can-begin-to-eat-better/

(4) https://www.cdc.gov/nchs/fastats/obesity-overweight.htm

(5) https://www.ncbi.nlm.nih.gov/pubmed/15523086

(6) https://www.ncbi.nlm.nih.gov/pubmed/18452640

(7) http://www.nejm.org/doi/10.1056/NEJMoa1501451

(8) https://www.iofbonehealth.org/facts-statistics

(9) https://newsroom.heart.org/news/magnesium-may-modestly-lower-blood-pressure

(10) https://www.ncbi.nlm.nih.gov/pmc/articles/PMC4549665/

(11) https://www.ncbi.nlm.nih.gov/pubmed/27910808

(12) https://www.ncbi.nlm.nih.gov/pmc/articles/PMC3024842/

(13) https://www.ncbi.nlm.nih.gov/pubmed/20329590

(14) https://www.ncbi.nlm.nih.gov/pmc/articles/PMC3335257/

(15) https://www.ncbi.nlm.nih.gov/pubmed/21864752

(16) https://www.ncbi.nlm.nih.gov/pmc/articles/PMC5133084/

(17) https://www.ncbi.nlm.nih.gov/pmc/articles/PMC2235907/

(18) https://www.health.harvard.edu/diseases-and-conditions/glycemic-index-and-glycemic-load-for-100-foods

(19) https://health.usnews.com/best-diet/dash-diet

(20) https://www.ncbi.nlm.nih.gov/pmc/articles/PMC1993964/

(21)https://jamanetwork.com/journals/jamainternalmedicine/fullarticle/414155

(22) https://www.cdc.gov/heartdisease/facts.htm

(23) https://www.ncbi.nlm.nih.gov/pubmed/21058045

(24)https://www.ncbi.nlm.nih.gov/pubmed/26622263

(25) https://www.ncbi.nlm.nih.gov/pubmed/23466047/

(26) https://www.ncbi.nlm.nih.gov/pmc/articles/PMC1402378/

(27) https://www.ncbi.nlm.nih.gov/pubmed/9927006

(28) https://www.ncbi.nlm.nih.gov/pubmed/27102172

(29) https://www.ncbi.nlm.nih.gov/pubmed/11283423

(30)
https://www.ncbi.nlm.nih.gov/pmc/articles/PMC2376744/

(31)
https://www.ncbi.nlm.nih.gov/pmc/articles/PMC4683169/